JUST A NURSE

Just A Nurse

FOR MY HUSBAND, JOHN, THANK YOU FOR BEING THERE DURING THESE TIMES; MY CHILDREN, BROCK, MOLLY AND EMMETT, SO THAT THEY UNDERSTAND SOME OF MOM'S EXPERIENCES AND MY JOYS NURSING; AND MY COLLEAGUES WHO WERE THERE WITH ME THROUGH IT ALL

Table Of Contents

A NOTE TO THE READER

THE STORIES SHARED IN THIS BOOK ARE BASED ON PERSONAL EXPERIENCES. I HAVE HAD MANY EXPERIENCES NURSING AND EACH OF THESE STORIES HAS AFFECTED MY PRACTICE IN ONE WAY OR ANOTHER FOR THE BETTER. THE NAMES OF THE CHARACTERS HAVE BEEN ALTERED TO SAVE THEIR IDENTITY AND MAINTAIN CONFIDENTIALITY.

A Borrowed Mother

The number one thing in nursing school I learned was that I must always be adaptable to any situation. I found myself in a very vulnerable profession that required all my holistic being to embrace all unexpected occurrences with a fearless face. This face, at this time was meant for two young children. I was working as a staff nurse on the hospice unit. This unit came with expected outcomes which were routinely the practice of end-of-life care for the patient and their families. This unit was such a blessing in my life, and I truly became the nurse I always wanted to be on this unit. I felt at home, and I thought I had found what I would enjoy doing for the rest of my life as a RN. One morning shift, I came onto the unit to find one of my patients had died in the early morning just a few hours ago. The woman was younger, in her mid-thirties, and was surrounded by those from her home community. I would be required to care for her body and move it to the morgue once her family and friends departed from the room. After collecting the information on the rest of the patients I would have that day, I was to report to the room of this woman and provide further instructions to her loved ones and my condolences. I moved a little slower than normal these days as I was pregnant with my second child, my daughter. I waddle down the hallway and before I can get to the entryway of the room, two young girls, not older than eight years old, come running out of the room. They run into my body and grasp onto my legs. My balance, though slightly off due to my womb, managed to not allow me to fall over. I froze. I look up at the family members, all men in the room, with tears in their eyes. One comes over to me and asks me, "Can they stay with you a while? We are waiting on her sister still". In absolute disbelief of what I am witnessing, I reply very quietly, "of course". He turns away and continues to comfort those with him. I remain in the hallway with the two little girls for what seems like an eternity, just sitting on the floor with them. I offer up two arms and they embrace with me. I sit in the quiet and let them cry and beg me to bring their mom back. I stroke their hair and rub their tears off their faces. Instinct kicks in and I begin to rock back and forth. I hum a random tune that to this day I cannot remember. One of the girls stops crying and says, "My mom sings, too".

I hear a voice of a woman calmly say, "Hi there, girls. Come with Auntie". The two girls get up and leave me. Her sister has arrived. The woman thanks us all for the wonderful care of her family. They all depart as expected, and my shift continues for the next ten hours. I have the best team working on hospice. They have divided up my load of patients and cared for them while I sat with the girls. I walk into the patient's room, smile at her and finish my care for her. I transport her to the morgue while humming that song and I know her little girls will be fine. This is one of my favourite moments of being Just a Nurse.

Just A Nurse

FOR THE LOVE OF AN ADDICT

I had not encountered a person with an addiction. Well, at least I thought I had not. I was working in the Correctional Services Department for the local jail when I met the boy that would change my understanding of people who have addictions and provide me with my first success story. I do not have very many of these big stories, but since this was the first, it has proven to be the most impact on my life. Working as a RN in a jail has given me the opportunity to work with one of the most vulnerable populations in Northwestern Ontario, Canada. I had recently started my career as a RN on staff at the Thunder Bay Jail. I met many inmates from all walks of life, and all are males as the facility is an all-male institution. One of the inmates came into custody and was severely withdrawing from a variety of opiates including the notorious Fentanyl that has plagued the streets of Thunder Bay. There have been more studies completed on the appropriate treatment of opiate addictions and the withdrawing stages; however, I met this individual (I will give him a false name of Nathan) during the peak point of time where monitoring and providing minimal treatment was offered. Please keep in mind this absolutely no fault of anyone, just simply current practices with the times. I provided Nathan with fluids and medications to prevent severe nausea and vomiting. I was intrigued by Nathan as he kept crying out, "Don't ever do it, it's not worth it, I need out". Here was a young man, in his mid-twenties, crying and laying on the floor literally shitting his pants and vomiting up bile, begging for the pain to end and I looked him in the eye, and I asked him, "Why?". A few days later, once

Nathan had sobered up and had some sleep, I was completing a medication round where he was living when he stated, "to feel happy". I stood there and I did not understand. He repeated himself only this time, he added, "you asked me why and the answer is to feel happy. I can escape everything with drugs. I can feel happy". I was shocked. I did not think he heard me when he was withdrawing. I did not believe he would remember me even being there giving him fluids and making sure he was eating and taking medications.

Weeks later, I learned that Nathan was having issues with other inmates and was moved into an area where he could be isolated for his safety. I honestly figured he had made some bad deals with drugs in jail and was hiding out. I learned during his time there, he had reconnected with his mother. One of the Correctional Officers stopped me on my way out as I had finished my shift. He informed me that a "special visitation" was happening that night and invited me to witness it. Normally, nurses keep distance from their patients. We feel this is an appropriate way to create a safe barrier. This evening, I jumped over that barrier. I put myself in a vulnerable place that I like to call "being a human being". I witnessed Nathan's mother come visit him for the first time in jail. I had never seen someone so happy to see their loved one. This was the case for both individuals involved. He smiled the entire time I saw him, and she was overjoyed at how well he looked. This was truly an eye-opening experience for me as a nurse. It gave me hope that if we provide our patients with a form of empathy or understanding, they will give us something to hope for, something that we can view as a success. Nathan was discharged from custody not long after the visit and on his way out he mentioned, "I am happy with my mom". I knew in that moment; I would never see him again. This is the greatest success story of every Correctional Nurse.

All Nurses Get Naked

Aging is a funny part of life. People often associate aging with events like dying, becoming grandparents, losing their spouse, or retirement. All of these events have real significance, and these events are seen as normal. But why does no one talk about the quirky things that nurses do as they age? As a nurse, I can assure you this profession comes with points of quirkiness and specific traits that can usually lead to conversations of "have you ever seen…" or "this one patient I had was crazy and …". We tend to compare our stories and education, but it's funny we don't discuss the common nursing traits of aging. What I have experienced in my short time as a RN is this: all nurses get naked as they age. It is a common statement among nurses that we tend to not be so concerned with whom is in the room when discussing a gross story or describing a specific traumatic event that can leave scars on most people mentally, especially as time goes on. We just tend to not care. We especially do not care about our clothing as we age.

One patient I had was an elderly woman who was awaiting long term care. She was a retired ER charge nurse. Her sense of humour was astounding as she would chime into random conversation with anyone who would listen. She enjoyed the company of people and of her books. I was working day shift one weekend when I noticed this patient, we will call her Mary, walking with her four wheeled walker through the hallway and down to the sunroom, which was lit by the morning sunrise, and she was completely naked. I panicked. I ran down the hallway and grabbed a towel on the cart. Bringing her the towel I said, "Mary, here you are dear. You must have forgotten your clothes this morning". Not missing a beat, Mary looked at me and smiled saying "Nope, just wanted to air out the girls and get a good tan". I laughed. I was so caught off guard by the statement and Mary kept walking along. I explained to her that Mr. Smith was also in the room and was a little embarrassed as he had not seen a naked woman in years. She politely responded, "Oh, its ok. I'm a nurse. I don't mind". Mary eventually agreed to wear a housecoat. I brought her a morning cup of tea and asked her lots of questions about nursing back in the earlier years. She explained, "That's why I like to be naked. All nurses do. We had to wear those tight white dresses and the hose, my goodness; those stockings were so tight your voice could change three octaves. It's always nice to come home, and just be free".

We can learn a lot from our senior staff members. Mary taught me to be comfortable in every situation. She taught me to be confident in myself and if I was not sure of the answer, I need only to go find one.

Just A Nurse

A Beautiful Death

I was caring for a patient and his family on a hospice unit. Their son was dying from an inoperable brain tumor. It was my second experience caring for a child who was terminally ill. I understood that this boy was technically an adult; however, a battle that could not be won had been occurring for him since he was only five years old. This frail body now lying in a hospital bed was surrounded by balloons and books and family. You would have thought it was a birthday party. I was working the morning shift and I walked into the room to greet his mother. I observed her sleeping with her son wrapped in her arms. He looked beautiful. He looked peaceful. I went closer the bed to discover he was dead. I performed my assessment to confirm my findings, and with a very soft voice, I whispered out loud "0703". It takes a lot to scare a nurse. It really takes a lot to scare a nurse working on a hospice unit. We greet death like it's an old friend instead of being fearful. The moment I finished my whisper, the mother of the boy calmly said with her eyes shut "630". I jumped. I did not realize she had been awake the entire time. She looked at me, tears in eyes, and calmly stated, "He died at 630. I was able to hold him and let him fall asleep. It was beautiful". I have never in my life cried with a patient. I have cried with their families. This was no different. I had just returned to work after giving birth to my first-born son. I stayed in that room with the mother, and we exchanged moments in our sons' lives. She told me he wanted to just "go to sleep" one night. She knew this was the night. Mothers tend to have that intuition about their children. I asked her if she needed anything else and she just said "Time. I would like to hold him for a little more time". I had no words. I exited the room and did what any other sensible RN does when we go into shock- I threw up. At least that time, I made it to the staff bathroom. This is one of my sad stories and yet, it is beautiful. The peace that was felt in that room that early morning is something I will never forget. It is such a privilege to be welcomed into a patient's life, no matter what part of the lifespan they are on, and allowed to provide care. This story is one that I tell over and over again for the purpose of proving that nurses can learn from their patients. This woman taught me how to see the most beautiful points in life and in death; providing one last wish for her son to die comforted in the arms of his mother and in peaceful silence was the best gift received. She taught me how to go on nursing and caring for young people and not being afraid that they may die. This brave young man wanted nothing more than the comfort of someone holding him as he died. I took that knowledge, and I continued my practice differently. I never left a room empty. I stayed with my patients while they died if no one was there. I remained present through all conversations, and I contributed more to non-verbal communication. I recognized that although I am just a nurse, I am the patient's greatest asset. I am their advocate and their confidant. I realized how important it is to be human and allow myself to cry with my patients and have real feelings with them present. This story is the one that shaped my practice and created a better nurse.

Just A Nurse

A Time to Teach

I discovered my love of teaching mid-way in my career. I wanted to shape students and create great nurses. I began teaching in clinical placements with the local university. I really enjoyed working with students. They are like sponges and have a vast knowledge of the current health care trends and practices. Truly, I have learned much from them.

My favourite thing to teach is communication. I find this an essential component in nursing. If you cannot communicate, you cannot nurse. It is an absolute dance. I took on teaching a lab course which revolved around therapeutic communication and relationship building with the patient. This was a first-year course. I entered the room to discover over thirty students looking back at me. I determined at that point; I had no idea what I was doing. How was I going to teach these people about communication and not allow them to fall asleep? I wanted to be interesting. I wanted to gain their attention. I just really wanted them not to walk out. I started off with the traditional "tell me about yourself" and "this is who I am "speeches only to discover they were just as nervous as I was. I asked the students questions a lot. I wanted to know what they thought about nursing and what they wanted to learn. One brave soul raised their hand and stated, "I just want to know what to say to an old person". I burst out laughing. I was not being mean, but rather I was intrigued. I was raised in a home with my grandparents. I never really had to think about communication with the elderly as they were a part of my everyday life. I asked the students how to communicate and they were silent. They simply had no idea.

I explained the importance of nonverbal communication. It is approximately 92% of all communication as learned in many textbooks around the world. I explained to the students this meant looking at someone when you are speaking and when they speak. I had an idea of how to teach the best communication skills known to anyone. I told the students that I would bring in a guest speaker. They were very excited. The following class, I walked in with a blonde girl. She was so tiny that she could not see over the podium. She was also only four years old. She sat on the stool at the front of the classroom and stared into the crowd with no fear. She wore pink. It was her favourite colour. Her first words to the class were "Hi. I'm Molly". The students looked puzzled and yet, happy. I explained to them that this was my daughter. If they could talk to her, they would have no issue talking to an elderly person. Often times we are intimidated by our senior citizens when really they are as polite, cognizant and blunt as that of a four year old. My students enjoyed their interviews with Molly (that alone should be a book) and left the class feeling a little more hopeful for their clinical placements. Weeks later, I would have a few of these students in my clinical placement in long term care. These students had no concerns or hesitations sitting down with patients and looking them in the eye at their level just to talk. They were ok with silence. They were ok to offer a snack. As a nurse, I have learned the importance of returning to childlike faith in humanity. I continue to teach my students in this way and my children continue to remind me the importance of this faith. This lesson has also made me realize that a student can become a leader for nursing staff. Nurses tend to forget where they start from much like I forgot starting from a home raised with people of all ages. Communication is our foundation. We must always build up from it.

TRY TO NOT SCARE THE NEW PEOPLE

One fascination of mine has always been psychogeriatric nursing. This is where you must be very flexible, very compassionate and have a keen eye and excellent reflexes. You never know when a commode is going to be flying across the hallway in your direction. I was working the night shift on a small unit filled with geriatric patients most of whom were diagnosed with dementia. I really loved my years here. I met lovely families, I enjoyed my time caring for these patients and my colleagues taught me how to best manage my time on shift and remain flexible for the unknown events that can happen. An example of an unknown event or unknown flying object can be as simple as a commode. A commode is the type of toilet that a nurse will use with their patient that cannot make it to the bathroom but can stand and sit with a one person assist. The idea is to provide them with dignity while being able to give modified independence for the daily living task of voiding or having a bowel movement. I was walking with a new hire down the hallway one night. They had just graduated and were eager to get settled into their new job on the front lines. This new grad was full of hope and desires to help those that were elderly and not always aware of their surroundings. Psychogeriatric nursing had been a dream of theirs for the last four years of schooling. As we were walking toward the nursing station, the new grad casually asked me "so, do you think it will be a calm evening? Will I be doing anything cool or is this the sleep shift?" Nothing could have prepared that new grad quite like a bedpan full of fresh urine and soggy toilet paper being thrown in front of them as we approached the staff room on the unit. She screamed and jumped back in disbelief of what had just happened. I must admit, I was surprised that it was just urine. Then, the commode flew at us. The lovely vessel was filled with diarrhea and no paper so that as it flew in front of our faces, it splashed onto my uniform. I turned towards the patient's doorway to see a little 98lb woman angry. She was calling out "you bitch! I'll get you with my cane I will! "Many other colourful names were called and the new hire vomited on floor in the hallway. I calmly asked Doris (yes, her name has been altered for the book) if she would like a snack, specifically two cookies with warm milk and she nodded to me "yeah and hurry up-waiting all day for my cookies." The frail woman walked to her bed and sat down glaring at the new hire. I told the new grad "This is why I keep an extra set of scrubs in my locker. Bathroom is over there, mop is in the closet, and yes, we will have some events tonight. It's a full moon. "

Doris was angry because she did not recognize the new person who entered the unit. She was scared. Her happiest memories were from childhood visits to her grandmothers where she always was allowed two cookies and a warm glass of milk. I introduced the new grad to Doris and explained that she would be working on the unit. Doris did not like change but accepted the cookies as a peace offering.

The importance of nursing and communication cannot be stressed enough. Calmness is essential. The new grad quickly learned that not every dementia case is the same. Every person we meet has a story and there always plot twists in your shift. Nursing has allowed me to become flexible. I have never forgotten this story. I will never look at a commode the same again.

TRUST YOUR GUT

I am just a nurse. I have the qualifications to provide a variety of care based on my skill set and never-ending education. This has come in handy while working in corrections. A new admission came into the jail I work at with an injury that was labelled as a stab wound. Now, what you are picturing is already incorrect. The wound was to the right inner bicep and was approximately 2cm x 0.5cm. At first glance, there was almost no indent. Further assessment proved approximately 1cm tunneling was present. The area was clean, no bleeding present and almost no redness. The young man was otherwise healthy and did not have a history of steady drug or alcohol use other than the weekend that had brought him here to the jail. It was still early in my shift. I was on a twelve-hour rotation and this was my final shift before two days off. He was my only admission that day. It seemed simple, but something deep in my gut told me to send this guy immediately to ER. Naturally, I did what any sensible nurse would do- I sent him to ER after an argument with the sergeant on duty and a few other Correctional Staff. I could not shake that feeling. It had been a few hours since I had sent the inmate when the officers escorting the inmate called the jail to let the sergeant know the inmate was being admitted to hospital for further treatment. I honestly could not believe it either when I heard the diagnosis of compartment syndrome. He remained in care at the hospital for several days and surgery took place. I remember being asked how I knew he was sick by a staff member, and I still have no idea. I chalk it up as a lucky guess.

Nursing school always tells of stories where nurses understand more than they should and can see a detrimental episode before it happens. They save lives. I do not see this in myself yet, but I have not ignored my gut instinct since this episode. Again, I am just a nurse.

Just A Nurse

No one can ever prepare you for nursing life. You become immersed in sensitive information given to you by strangers. Permission is granted to you to perform tasks on people that don't know you can't remember your name and have no choice but to have trust in everything you do. You are held high as heroes by some and spat on by most. Your language must change to best suit your patient. You have limited time to attend to all their needs and you will be criticized on how well you make a bed. The people that will always judge you the most are your peers. Nurses are ruthless and known to "eat their young". We are taught this in school. We are taught this in clinical. We say this to new hires and new grads. I never did believe that a fear tactic worked, but I do believe in respect. I have gained more knowledge and practical skills from my peers than anyone. I have had nurses call me "useless", "replaceable", "stupid" and even "lazy". I have fought with co-workers over proper documentation and time management. I have witnessed the growth of a new manager. I have cared for my dying colleague and wrapped my arms around my fellow weeping peers as we say goodbye. I have learned that every nurse is different. Every nurse has a very special and specific skill that they bring to the team. I have worked in settings where multiple nurses have the same skill and it will not always be easy to work with, but we manage. We care for each other. We look out for each other, and we argue like family does. I currently work in a setting that believes in the saying "I got your back". This group is interesting. It has changed. It has developed into a new family. I know every day I go to work, and I will be safe because my nursing family is there. No matter what happens, they will be there. Some of the present skill sets that encompass my nursing family are the ability to remain calm, the ability to multitask, the ability to document precisely and with such detail you can visualize what happened, the veteran with the most knowledge from several areas of practice, the ability to describe and understand feelings and the ability to be comfortable. It is important to also recognize that nursing teams incorporate other professions like physicians, nurse practitioners, social workers, and secretaries. Everyone knows they have a place and a purpose, or the team fails.

Jail nursing has proven that team approach is important. We all need each other, or we fail. Sometimes, we forget this, and it shows, but we never stop connecting. Nurses are usually empaths by nature. We share the common statement "I love you" more frequently in this higher risk setting than anywhere else I have ever worked. It shows. It matters. I sometimes believe I am just a nurse. The bonus in this family; they are with me no matter what happens until I have my "sentence satisfied".